FEELING PINK

Comforting, Cozy, and Cheerful Words

for Breast Cancer Survivors

by: Torran Bagamary and Michelle Iglesias

CCC Books

PO Box 1827

Westfield, MA 01086

by: Torran Bagamary and Michelle Iglesias

Copyright © 2008 CCC Books

Published in the U.S.A. by CCC Books

PO Box 1827, Westfield, MA 01086

(413) 205-8346

www.stillbeautifulstore.com

ISBN # 978-0-578-00801-1

In memory of Michael B. Lynn

and his three loving dogs,

Chewy, Chuck, and Chico

CONTENTS

INTRODUCTION

Every survivor can use a few words of encouragement during treatment and recovery. The journey toward healing and recuperation can be emotionally and physically draining. This book is a lovely treasure trove of inspiring and uplifting quotes, perfect for revitalizing any survivor's heart, head, health, and happiness. Reading a few pages from this book will improve your mood and attitude, reduce stress and anxiety, and aid in coping and adjusting with the changes that you face. No one has to go through this alone and we could all use a little spiritual guidance. This book will help you on your way to recovery.

Michelle Iglesias
Wilbraham, Massachusetts
4 year survivor

HONOR

Accepting, Respecting, and Loving Yourself

A cancer survivor said to me once, "Scars are just a reminder of the battle we fought…a symbol of strength and courage we can see every day." Indeed, this is true. You were both strong and brave in your fight against breast cancer. You are a victorious survivor. There is much to be honored in this achievement. Accept yourself, respect yourself, and love yourself.

Love yourself unconditionally,

just as you love those closest to you despite their faults.

Les Brown

Self-respect permeates every aspect of your life.

Joe Clark

Life is a struggle, accept it.

Mother Teresa

Acceptance of what has happened is the first step

to overcoming the consequences of any misfortune.

William James

But there isn't any second half of myself

waiting to plug in and make me whole.

It's there. I'm already whole.

Sally Field

The first step toward change is awareness.

The second step is acceptance.

Nathaniel Branden

Respect your efforts, respect yourself.

Self-respect leads to self-discipline.

When you have both firmly under your belt,

that's real power.

Clint Eastwood

Accept yourself as you are.

Otherwise you will never see opportunity.

You will not feel free to move toward it;

you will feel you are not deserving.

Maxwell Maltz

Self-respect is the cornerstone of all virtue.

John Herschel

I celebrate myself, and sing myself.

Walt Whitman

Resolve to be thyself: and know,

that he who finds himself,

loses his misery.

Matthew Arnold

Do not wish to be anything except what you are.

Saint Francis De Sales

When you feel good about yourself,

others will feel good about you, too.

Jake Steinfeld

The first step toward change is acceptance.

Once you accept yourself,

you open the door to change.

That's all you have to do.

Change is not something you do,

it's something you allow.

Will Garcia

Self-love is the greatest of all flatters.

Francois de la Rochefoucauld

The quickest way to change your attitude toward pain

is to accept the fact that everything that happens to us

has been designed for our spiritual growth.

M. Scott Peck

Serenity comes when you trade

expectations for acceptance.

Anonymous

Once we accept our limits,

we go beyond them.

Brendan Francis

You have to accept whatever comes

and the only important thing is that you meet it

with courage and with the best that you have to give.

Eleanor Roosevelt

Our entire life consists ultimately in

accepting ourselves as we are.

Jean Anouilh

When you accept the ill befallen,

the process of healing has begun.

Anonymous

If I could define enlightenment briefly

I would say it is

'the quiet acceptance of what is'.

Dr. Wayne Dyer

Don't forget to love yourself.

Soren Kierkegaard

Self acceptance is

the freedom to see oneself without denial.

Nathaniel Branden

We cannot change anything until we accept it.

Condemnation does not liberate, it oppresses.

Carl Gustav Jung

You yourself, as much as anybody in the entire universe,

deserve your love & affection.

Buddha

Everything in life depends

on how that life accepts its limits.

James Baldwin

Happiness can exist only in acceptance.

Denis De Rougamont

Love yourself first and everything else falls into line.

You really have to love yourself

to get anything done in this world.

Lucille Ball

Accept everything about yourself – I mean everything,

you are you and that is the beginning and the end –

no apologies, no regrets.

Clark Moustakes

The most terrifying thing

is to accept oneself completely.

Carl Gustav Jung

There comes a time when you have to stand up and shout:

This is me damn it! I look the way I look,

think the way I think, feel the way I feel,

love the way I love! I am a whole complex package.

Take me... or leave me. Accept me – or walk away!

Do not try to make me feel like less of a person,

just because I don't fit your idea of who I should be

and don't try to change me to fit your mold.

If I need to change, I alone will make that decision.

When you are strong enough to love yourself 100%,

good and bad – you will be amazed

at the opportunities that life presents you.

Stacey Charter

If I despised myself,

it would be no compensation if everyone saluted me,

and if I respect myself,

it does not trouble me if others hold me lightly.

Max Nordau

Understanding is the first step to acceptance,

and only with acceptance can there be recovery.

Joanne Kathleen Rowling

For after all,

the best thing one can do when it's raining

is to let it rain.

Henry Wadsworth Longfellow

Accepting does not necessarily mean

'liking,' 'enjoying,' or 'condoning.' I can accept what is –

and be determined to evolve from there.

It is not acceptance but denial that leaves me stuck.

Nathaniel Branden

Lord grant me

the serenity to accept the things I cannot change,

the courage to change the things I can,

and the wisdom to know the difference.

Saint Francis of Assisi

Self-respect knows no considerations.

Mahatma Gandhi

Some people confuse acceptance with apathy,

but there's all the difference in the world.

Apathy fails to distinguish between

what can and what cannot be helped;

acceptance makes that distinction.

Apathy paralyzes the will-to-action;

acceptance frees it by relieving it of impossible burdens.

Arthur Gordon

The way I see it, if you want the rainbow,

you gotta put up with the rain.

Dolly Parton

Acceptance is not submission;

it is acknowledgement of the facts of a situation.

Then deciding what you're going to do about it.

Kathleen Casey Theisen

Self-love is the instrument

of our preservation.

Voltaire

We must accept life for what it actually is –

a challenge to our quality without which

we should never know of what stuff we are made,

or grow to our full stature.

Ida R. Wylie

When you're a beautiful person on the inside,

there is nothing in the world

that can change that about you…

If you can't accept yourself,

then certainly no one else will.

Sasha Azevedo

How little a thing can make us happy

when we feel that we have earned it.

Mark Twain

Everything in life that we really accept

undergoes a change.

Katherine Mansfield

Acceptance of one's life has nothing to do with resignation;

it does not mean running away from the struggle.

On the contrary, it means accepting it as it comes,

with all the handicaps of heredity, of suffering,

of psychological complexes and injustices.

Dr. Paul Tournier

He that respects himself is safe from others;

he wears a coat of mail that none can pierce.

Henry Wadsworth Longfellow

Our entire life,

with our fine moral code and our precious freedom,

consists ultimately in accepting ourselves as we are.

Jean Anouilh

Self acceptance comes from

meeting life's challenges vigorously.

Don't numb yourself to your trials and difficulties,

nor build mental walls to exclude pain from your life.

You will find peace not by trying to escape your problems,

but by confronting them courageously.

You will find peace not in denial, but in victory.

J. Donald Walters

Of all afflictions, the worst is self-contempt.

Berthold Auerbach

The curious paradox is that

when I accept myself just as I am,

then I can change.

Carl Rogers

My imperfections and failures

are as much a blessing from God

as my successes and my talents

and I lay them both at his feet.

Mahatma Gandhi

Our first and last love is – self-love.

Christian Bovee

There is a voice inside which speaks and says:

'This is the real me!'

William James

HEAD

Gaining Confidence and Self-Esteem

Adjusting to limitations from surgery and treatment can be difficult for any cancer survivor. The inability to perform certain tasks as he or she once was can lower a cancer victim's sense of worth. A fellow survivor said to me once, "If you can no longer run, it's because you are meant to walk." The message is an important one – that all survivors should be confident in the things he or she can do. Don't let physical restrictions hold you back. Believe in yourself, be confident in yourself, and make the most of what you have.

You are what you think.

You are what you go for.

You are what you do.

Bob Richards

Whether you think you can or think you can't –

you are right.

Henry Ford

Problems are only opportunities in work clothes.

Henry J. Kaiser

Nothing builds self-esteem and self-confidence

like accomplishment.

Thomas Carlyle

The will to do

springs from the knowledge that we can do.

James Allen

Trust yourself,

then you will know how to live.

Johann Wolfgang von Goethe

Whatever good things we build

end up building us.

Jim Rohn

To establish true self-esteem

we must concentrate on our successes

and forget about the failures and the negatives in our lives.

Denis Waitley

Self-pity gets you nowhere.

Harry Emerson Fosdick

Self-respect permeates every aspect of your life.

Joe Clark

The best way to gain self-confidence

is to do what you are afraid to do.

Anonymous

What a man thinks of himself,

that is which determines, or rather indicates his fate.

Henry David Thoreau

The man who acquires the ability

to take full possession of his own mind

may take possession of anything else to which

he is justly entitled.

Andrew Carnegie

A man cannot be comfortable

without his own approval.

Mark Twain

Accept that you are enough.

You don't need to be anything that you are not.

Dr. Wayne Dyer

If we really love ourselves,

everything in our life works.

Louise L. Hay

I am an artist of my own creation.

I like myself.

Sondra Ray

The way you treat yourself sets the standard for others.

Sonya Friedman

If you put a small value on yourself,

rest assured that the world will not raise your price.

Anonymous

First thing every morning before you arise say out loud,

"I believe", three times.

Norman Vincent Peale

The most important key

to the permanent enhancement of self-esteem

is the practice of positive inner-talk.

Denis Waitley

No one can make you feel inferior

without your permission.

Eleanor Roosevelt

Of all the judgment we pass in life,

none is more important

than the judgment we pass on ourselves.

Nathaniel Branden

What lies behind us and what lies ahead of us

are tiny matters compared to what lives within us.

Ralph Waldo Emerson

Too many people overvalue what they are not

and undervalue what they are.

Malcolm S. Forbes

Opportunities to find deeper powers within ourselves

come when life seems most challenging.

Joseph Campbell

Know yourself

and you will win all battles.

Sun Tzu

Our strength often increases in proportion

to the obstacles imposed upon it.

Paul De Rapin

People are like stained-glass windows.

They sparkle and shine when the sun is out,

but when the darkness sets in

their true beauty is revealed

only if there is light from within.

Elisabeth Kübler-Ross

The stars are constantly shining,

but often we do not see them until the dark hours.

Earl Riney

Knock the 't' off the 'can't'.

Samuel Johnson

For real self-esteem is not derived from

the great things you've done, the things you won.

The mark you've made –

but an appreciation of yourself for what you are.

Maxwell Max

Once we believe in ourselves, we can risk curiosity,

wonder, spontaneous delight, or any experience

that reveals the human spirit.

E. E. Cummings

A person's worth in this world is estimated

according to the value they put on themselves.

Jean de La Bruyere

Every new adjustment is a crisis in self-esteem.

Eric Hoffer

Put all excuses aside and remember this:

YOU are capable.

Zig Ziglar

Self-pity is our worst enemy

and if we yield to it,

we can never do anything wise in the world.

Helen Keller

The average estimate themselves

by what they do,

the above average

by what they are.

Johann Friedrich Von Schiller

HEART

Continuing to Grow and Follow Your Dreams

With every beat, your heart is reminding you of your survival. Now, more than ever, your heart should continue to remain strong while spirits and emotions are drained. Your heart holds the willingness and determination to make the best of your life. It's time to follow your heart, learn from this experience, and make your life fulfilling.

The most important thing in illness is never to lose heart.

Nikolai Lenin

You can do anything in life you set your mind to,

provided it is powered by your heart.

Doug Firebaugh

My mind tells me to give up,

but my heart won't let me.

Anonymous

When your heart is in your dreams,

no request is too extreme.

Jiminy Cricket

My eyes are an ocean in which

my dreams are reflected.

Anna M. Uhlich

A kind heart is a foundation of gladness,

making everything in its vicinity freshen into smiles.

Washington Irving

Empty pockets never held anyone back.

Only empty heads and empty hearts can do that.

Norman Vincent Peale

A light heart lives long.

William Shakespeare

Our heart carries the wings of our dreams

and the desire to realize them.

Fernando Soave

We should show life neither as it is

or as it ought to be,

but only as we see it in our dreams.

Leo Tolstoy

Recognize that you have the courage within you

to fulfill the purpose of your birth.

Summon forth the power of your inner courage

and live the life of your dreams.

Gurumayi Chidvilasananda

Perhaps it's good to have a beautiful mind,

but an even greater gift is to have a beautiful heart.

John Nash

Dream as if you'll live forever,

live as if you'll die today.

James Dean

The most powerful agent of growth and transformation

is something much more basic than any technique:

a change of heart.

John Welwood

Dreams are renewable.

No matter what our age or condition,

there are still untapped possibilities within us

and new beauty waiting to be born.

Dr. Dale E. Turner

It is essential to our well-being, and to our lives,

that we play and enjoy life.

Every single day do something that makes your heart sing.

Marcia Wieder

It may be that those who do most, dream most.

Stephen Butler Leacock

Our sweetest experiences of affection

are meant to point us to that realm which is

the real and endless home of the heart.

Henry Ward Beecher

All that is worth cherishing

begins in the heart, not the head.

Suzanne Chapin

Great hearts steadily send forth the secret forces that

incessantly draw great events.

Ralph Waldo Emerson

A person's world is only as big as their heart.

Tanya A. Moore

The greatest treasures are those

invisible to the eye

but found by the heart.

Anonymous

When your heart begins to tell you things

that your mind does not,

then you are getting the Spirit of the Lord.

Harold B. Lee

Within your heart, keep one still, secret spot

where dreams may go.

Louise Driscoll

Every great achievement is the victory

of a flaming heart.

Ralph Waldo Emerson

It is the heart that makes a man rich.

He is rich according to what he is,

not according to what he has.

Henry Ward Beecher

Your work is to discover your world

and then with all your heart

give yourself to it.

Buddha

Follow your heart, but be quiet for a while first.

Ask questions, then feel the answer.

Learn to trust your heart.

Anonymous

Wherever you go, go with all your heart.

Confucius

Man, alone, has the power to

transform his thoughts into physical reality;

man, alone, can dream

and make his dreams come true.

Napoleon Hill

A merry heart is like medicine for the soul.

Joyce C. Lock

A joyful heart is the inevitable result

of a heart burning with love.

Mother Teresa

Hold fast to dreams, for if dreams die,

life is a broken winged bird that cannot fly.

Lanston Hughes

If I keep a green bough in my heart,

then the singing bird will come.

Chinese Proverb

Great beauty, great strength, and great riches

are really and truly of no great use;

a right heart exceeds all.

Benjamin Franklin

The heart has reasons

that reason does not understand.

Jacques Benigne Bossuel

Write it on your heart

that every day is the best day of the year.

Ralph Waldo Emerson

In prayer it is better to have a heart without words

than words without a heart.

Mahatma Gandhi

A kind heart is a fountain of gladness,

making everything in its vicinity

freshen into smiles.

Washington Irving

You change your life by changing your heart.

Anonymous

Where your pleasure is, there is your treasure:

where your treasure, there your heart;

where your heart, there your happiness.

Saint Augustine

Yesterday is but a vision,

and tomorrow is only a dream.

But today well-lived

makes every yesterday a dream of happiness,

and every tomorrow a dream of hope.

Anonymous

The greatest test of courage on earth

is to bear defeat without losing heart.

Robert Ingersoll

The best and most beautiful things in the world

cannot be seen or even touched.

They must be felt with the heart.

Helen Keller

Your heart will not lie to you,

as long as you tell it the truth.

Michelle C. Ustaszeski

Tears are the safety valve of the heart when

too much pressure is laid on it.

Albert Smith

Only do what your heart tells you.

Princess Diana

Tell your heart that the fear of suffering

is worse than the suffering itself.

And no heart has ever suffered

when it goes in search of its dream.

Paulo Coelho

There is a light that shines beyond all things on earth,

beyond the highest, the very highest heavens.

This is the light that shines in your heart.

Chandogya Upanished

Go confidently in the direction of your dreams.

Live the life you have imagined.

Henry David Thoreau

Nothing is impossible to a valiant heart.

Jeanne D'Albret

Who looks outside, dreams;

who looks inside, awakens.

Carl Gustav Jung

Keep your feet on the ground,

but let your heart soar as high as it will.

A.W. Tozer

Our truest life is when we are in dreams awake.

Henry David Thoreau

It is not the size of a man

but the size of his heart that matters.

Evander Holyfield

In a full heart there is room for everything,

and in an empty heart there is room for nothing.

Antonio Porchia

If wrinkles must be written upon our brow,

let them not be written upon the heart;

the spirit should not grow old.

James A. Garfield

Follow your heart

and your dreams will come true.

Anonymous

The only lasting beauty

is the beauty of the heart.

Rumi

The future belongs to those

who believe in the beauty of their dreams.

Eleanor Roosevelt

Dreams are the touchstones of our character.

Henry David Thoreau

If you can imagine it, you can create it.

If you can dream it, you can become it.

William Arthur Ward

Hope is the dream of the waking man.

French Proverb

To unpathed waters,

undreamed shores.

William Shakespeare

Life is a cup

to be filled not drained.

Anonymous

You see things;

and you say "Why?"

But I dream things that never were;

and I say "Why not?"

George Bernard Shaw

Keep your heart open to dreams.

For as long as there's a dream, there is hope,

and as long as there is hope,

there is joy in living.

Anonymous

HEALTH

Developing Strength of Body, Mind, and Soul

Various types of surgeries and treatments, and other factors such as age, and prior health issues, make the road to recovery different for each survivor. Yet, everyone can feel healthy once again—body, mind, and soul. The healing process takes time and patience, and a willingness to make the necessary changes in your life that will lead to a healthy, complete, you.

From the bitterness of disease

man learns the sweetness of health.

Catalan Proverb

Gold that buys health can never be ill spent.

Thomas Dekker

When praying for healing, ask great things of God

and expect great thing from God.

But let us seek for that healing that really matters,

the healing of the heart, enabling us to trust God simply,

face God honestly, and live triumphantly.

Arlo F. Newell

The hardest thing you can do is smile

when you are ill, in pain, or depressed.

But this no-cost remedy is a necessary first half-step

if you are to start on the road to recovery.

Allen Klein

It is health that is real wealth and not

pieces of gold and silver.

Mahatma Gandhi

To insure good health:

eat lightly, breath deeply, live moderately,

cultivate cheerfulness, and maintain an interest in life.

William Londen

Know, then, whatever cheerful and serene supports the mind

supports the body too.

John Armstrong

Forgiveness is the way to true health and happiness.

Gerald Jampolsky

Health is the condition of wisdom,

and the sign is cheerfulness –

an open and noble temper.

Ralph Waldo Emerson

Healing in its fullest sense requires

looking into our heart and expanding our awareness

of who we are.

Mitchell Gaynor

Our greatest healer is sitting right under our nose,

moving in and out – our breath.

Jacquelyn Small

Health is a state of complete physical,

mental and social well-being,

and not merely the absence

of disease or infirmity.

World Health Organization

The power of love to change bodies is legendary,

built into folklore, common sense, and everyday experience.

Love moves the flesh, it pushes matter around....

Throughout history, "tender loving care" has uniformly been

recognized as a valuable element in healing.

Larry Dossey

He who takes medicine and neglects to diet

wastes the skill of his doctors.

Chinese Proverb

He who has health, has hope.

And he who has hope, has everything.

Arabian Proverb

Being in a good frame of mind

helps keep one in the picture of health.

Anonymous

The trouble with always trying to preserve

the health of the body is that it is so difficult to do

without destroying the health of the mind.

G.K. Chesterton

The secret of health for both mind and body

is not to mourn the past,

nor to worry about the future,

but to live the present moment wisely and earnestly.

Buddha

Fall seven times,

stand up eight.

Japanese Proverb

Diseases of the soul are more dangerous

and more numerous than those of the body.

Cicero

Sickness comes on horseback

but departs on foot.

Dutch Proverb

The power to heal is in you…

Andrew Weil

In order to change we must be sick and tired

of being sick and tired.

Anonymous

A good laugh and a long sleep

are the best cures in the doctor's book.

Irish Proverb

The appearance of a disease is swift as an arrow;

its disappearance slow, like a thread.

Chinese Proverb

A healthy body and soul come from

an unencumbered mind and body.

Ymber Delecto

The healthy, the strong individual,

is the one who asks for help when he needs it.

Whether he has an abscess on his knees or in his soul.

Rona Barrett

The best and most efficient pharmacy

is within your own system.

Robert C. Peale

My own prescription for health

is less paperwork and more running barefoot

through the grass.

Leslie Grimutter

Health is a state of complete harmony

of the body, mind and spirit.

When one is free from physical disabilities and mental

distractions, the gates of the soul open.

B.K.S. Iyengar

Health is like money,

we never have a true idea of its value until we lose it.

Josh Billings

Our body is a machine for living.

It is organized for that, it is its nature.

Let life go on in it unhindered and let it defend itself,

it will do more than if you paralyze it

by encumbering it with remedies.

Leo Tolstoy

Health and cheerfulness

naturally beget each other.

Joseph Addison

When an illness knocks you on your ass,

you should stay down and relax for a while

before trying to get back up.

Candea Core-Starke

Health is not simply the absence of sickness.

Hannah Green

A wise man should consider that health

is the greatest of human blessings,

and learn how by his own thought

to derive benefit from his illnesses.

Hippocrates

Confidence and hope do more good than physic.

Galen

Everyone who is born holds dual citizenship,

in the kingdom of the well and in the kingdom of the sick.

Although we all prefer to use only the good passport,

sooner or later each of us is obliged, at least for a spell,

to identify ourselves as citizens of that other place.

Susan Sontag

Hear your heart. Heart your health.

Faith Seehill

Pain (any pain--emotional, physical, mental) has a message.

The information it has about our life

can be remarkably specific, but it usually falls

into one of two categories:

"We would be more alive if we did more of this," and,

"Life would be more lovely if we did less of that."

Once we get the pain's message,

and follow its advice,

the pain goes away.

Peter McWilliams

It's no coincidence

that four of the six letters in health are "heal."

Ed Northstrum

Health is not valued till sickness comes.

Dr. Thomas Fuller

It is amazing how much crisper

the general experience of life becomes

when your body is given a chance

to develop a little strength.

Frank Duff

The more severe the pain or illness,

the more severe will be the necessary changes.

These may involve breaking bad habits,

or acquiring some new and better ones.

Peter McWilliams

Courage consists in the power of self-recovery.

Ralph Waldo Emerson

Love is a mutual self-giving

which ends in self-recovery.

Fulton J. Sheen

It does not matter how deep you fall,

what matters is how high you bounce back.

Anonymous

Determination, patience and courage

are the only things needed to improve any situation.

Peter Sinclair

One of the most sublime experiences we can ever have

is to wake up feeling healthy after we have been sick.

Rabbi Harold Kushner

Make your own recovery

the first priority in your life.

Robin Norwood

Health of body and mind is a great blessing,

if we can bear it.

John Henry Cardinal Newman

While we may not be able to control

all that happens to us,

we can control

what happens inside us.

Benjamin Franklin

How sickness enlarges the dimension

of a man's self to himself!

Charles Lamb

Superman's not brave.

You can't be brave if you're indestructible.

It's every day people, like you and me,

that are brave knowing we could easily

be defeated but still continue forward.

Anonymous

Health is a large word.

It embraces not the body only,

but the mind and spirit as well;...

and not today's pain or pleasure alone,

but the whole being and outlook of a man.

James H. West

HOPE

Cultivating Optimism and Faith

Hope breeds positive thinking. You must believe that brighter days lay ahead. Doubt, fear, anger, or any other negative emotion, will only prevent you from making positive changes in your life. If you want the best for yourself, you have to hope for it. Think positively; and make the best of this experience.

Your living is determined

not so much by what life brings to you

as by the attitude you bring to life;

not so much by what happens to you

as by the way your mind looks at what happens.

Kahlil Gibran

He who has faith has...

an inward reservoir of courage, hope, confidence,

calmness, and assuring trust that all will come out well –

even though to the world it may appear

to come out most badly.

B.C. Forbes

Faith is the substance of things hoped for,

the evidence of things not seen.

Bible

To be upset over what you don't have

is to waste what you do have.

Ken S. Keyes

Things turn out best for the people who make the best

out of the way things turn out.

Art Linkletter

If we shall take the good we find, asking no questions,

we shall have heaping measures.

Ralph Waldo Emerson

Hope is the physician of each misery.

Irish Proverb

Hope is necessary in every condition.

The miseries of poverty, sickness, of captivity,

would, without this comfort, be insupportable.

Samuel Johnson

Could we change our attitude,

we should not only see life differently,

but life itself would come to be different.

Katherine Mansfield

Hope is the word which God has written

on the brow of every man.

Victor Hugo

Hope is the only bee that makes honey without flowers.

Robert Ingersoll

A happy person is not a person

in a certain set of circumstances,

but rather a person

with a certain set of attitudes.

Hugh Downs

Hope is like a bird that senses the dawn

and carefully starts to sing while it is still dark.

Anonymous

Too many people miss the silver lining

because they're expecting gold.

Maurice Setter

But groundless hope, like unconditional love,

is the only kind worth having.

John Perry Barlow

In the night of death, hope sees a star,

and listening love can hear the rustle of a wing.

Robert Ingersoll

The person who sends out positive thoughts

activates the world around him positively

and draws back to himself positive results.

Norman Vincent Peale

Turn your face to the sun

and the shadows fall behind you.

Maori Proverb

People are not disturbed by things,

but by the view they take of them.

Epictetus

We plant seeds that will flower

as results in our lives,

so best to remove the weeds

of anger, avarice, envy and doubt...

Dorothy Day

Faith is putting all your eggs in God's basket,

then counting your blessings before they hatch.

Ramona C. Carroll

A positive attitude is not a destination.

It is a way of life.

Anonymous

Faith is the bird that sings when the dawn is still dark.

Rabindranath Tagore

I am an optimist.

It does not seem too much use being anything else.

Winston Churchill

You've gotta have hope.

Without hope life is meaningless.

Without hope life is meaning less and less.

Anonymous

The miserable have no other medicine.

But only hope.

William Shakespeare

Faith consists in believing when it is

beyond the power of reason to believe.

It is not enough that a thing be possible

for it to be believed.

Voltaire

Hope is patience with the lamp lit.

Tertullian

Wherever you go,

no matter what the weather,

always bring your own sunshine.

Anthony J. D'Angelo

Once you choose hope,

anything's possible.

Christopher Reeve

The human spirit is stronger

than anything that can happen to it.

C.C. Scott

Feed your faith

and your fears will starve to death.

Anonymous

Hope is like a road in the country;

there was never a road,

but when many people walk on it,

the road comes into existence.

Lin Yutang

In the depth of winter I finally learned that

there was in me an invincible summer.

Albert Camus

We must accept finite disappointment,

but we must never lose infinite hope.

Martin Luther King

Hope is the feeling we have

that the feeling we have is not permanent.

Mignon McLaughlin

If you don't like something change it;

if you can't change it,

change the way you think about it.

Mary Engelbreit

Let us rise up and be thankful,

for if we didn't learn a lot today,

at least we learned a little,

and if we didn't learn a little, at least we didn't get sick,

and if we got sick, at least we didn't die;

so, let us all be thankful.

Buddha

I always plucked a thistle and planted a flower

where I thought a flower would grow.

Abraham Lincoln

Every day may not be good,

but there's something good in every day.

Anonymous

I don't think of all the misery

but of the beauty that still remains.

Anne Frank

The block of granite which was an obstacle

in the pathway of the weak, became a stepping-stone

in the pathway of the strong.

Thomas Carlyle

Hope is putting faith to work

when doubting would be easier.

Anonymous

Whenever you fall,

pick something up.

Oswald Avery

Hope is faith holding out its hand in the dark.

George Iles

The greatest discovery of my generation

is that a human being can alter his life

by altering his attitudes.

William James

It's a lot better to hope than not to.

Benjamin J. Stein

Keep your face to the sunshine

and you cannot see the shadow.

It's what sunflowers do.

Helen Keller

Learn from yesterday,

live for today,

hope for tomorrow.

Anonymous

While there's life,

there's hope.

Roman Saying

The important thing is not

that we can live on hope alone,

but that life is not worth living without it.

Harvey Milk

Things never go so well

that one should have no fear,

and never so ill

that one should have no hope.

Turkish proverb

Hope is the thing with feathers that perches in the soul,

and sings the tunes without the words and never stops at all.

Emily Dickinson

Hope sees the invisible,

feels the intangible,

and achieves the impossible.

Anonymous

Attitude is a little thing

that makes a big difference.

Winston Churchill

Hope springs eternal in the human breast.

Alexander Pope

Faith is believing in things

when common sense tells you not to.

George Seaton

In all pleasures hope is a considerable part.

Samuel Johnson

Fear knocked at the door.

Faith answered.

And lo, no one was there.

Anonymous

I had the blues because I had no shoes

until upon the street,

I met a man who had no feet.

Persian Saying

Oh, my friend,

it's not what they take away from you that counts.

It's what you do with what you have left.

Hubert Humphrey

You must start with a positive attitude

or you will surely end without one.

Carrie Latet

Faith makes things possible,

not easy.

Anonymous

Blessed is he who expects nothing,

for he shall never be disappointed.

Benjamin Franklin

Faith is a passionate intuition.

William Wordsworth

Just because you're miserable

doesn't mean you can't enjoy your life.

Annette Goodheart

We cannot direct the wind

but we can adjust the sails.

Anonymous

In faith there is enough light

for those who want to believe

and enough shadows to blind

those who don't.

Blaise Pascal

Physical strength is measured

by what we can carry;

spiritual by what we can bear.

Anonymous

Positive anything is better

than negative thinking.

Elbert Hubbard

Optimism is the foundation of courage.

Nicholas Murray Butler

The Kingdom of Heaven is not a place,

but a state of mind.

John Burroughs

Faithless is he that says farewell

when the road darkens.

J.R.R. Tolkien

Attitude – not aptitude –

determines your altitude.

Anonymous

Positive thinking won't let you do anything

but it will let you do everything better than

negative thinking will.

Zig Ziglar

Faith is like radar

that sees through the fog.

Corrie Ten Boom

An optimist is the human personification of spring.

Susan J. Bissonette

Those who wish to sing,

always find a song.

Swedish Proverb

If an optimist had his left arm chewed off by an alligator,

he might say, in a pleasant and hopeful voice,

"Well, this isn't too bad.

I don't have my left arm anymore,

but at least nobody will ever ask me whether

I am right-handed or left-handed,"

but most of us would say something

more along the lines of

"Aaaaah! My arm! My arm!"

Lemony Snicket

No life is so hard

that you can't make it easier

by the way you take it.

Ellen Glasgow

Be like the bird that,

passing on her flight awhile on boughs too slight,

feels them give way beneath her, and yet sings,

knowing that she hath wings.

Victor Hugo

Some days there won't be a song in your heart.

Sing anyway.

Emory Austin

Reason is our soul's left hand,

Faith her right.

John Donne

He can who thinks he can,

and he can't who thinks he can't.

Orison Swett Marden

Faith can move mountains,

but don't be surprised if God

hands you a shovel.

Anonymous

Our attitudes control our lives.

Attitudes are a secret power

working twenty-four hours a day, for good or bad.

It is of paramount importance that we know

how to harness and control this great force.

Tom Blandi

Faith is reason grown courageous.

Sherwood Eddy

When the world says, "Give up,"

Hope whispers,

"Try it one more time."

Anonymous

Life is a shipwreck but we must not forget

to sing in the lifeboats.

Voltaire

Say you are well, or all is well with you,

And God shall hear your words

and make them true.

Ella Wheeler Wilcox

Man is a creature of hope and invention,

both of which belie the idea that things cannot be changed.

Tom Clancy

Hope is grief's best music.

Anonymous

Henceforth I ask not good-fortune,

I myself am good-fortune.

Walt Whitman

Hope is that thing with feathers

that perches in the soul

and sings the tune without the words

and never stops... at all.

Emily Dickinson

Since the house is on fire let us warm ourselves.

Italian Proverb

Faith makes the discords of the present

the harmonies of the future.

Robert Collyer

There are souls in this world which have the gift

of finding joy everywhere and

of leaving it behind them when they go.

Frederick Faber

A little faith will bring your soul to heaven,

but a lot of faith will bring heaven to your soul.

Anonymous

Hope begins in the dark,

the stubborn hope that if you just show up

and try to do the right thing,

the dawn will come.

Anne Lamott

Faith is taking the first step

even when you don't see the whole staircase.

Martin Luther King Jr

As your faith is strengthened you will find

that there is no longer the need to have a sense of control,

that things will flow as they will,

and that you will flow with them,

to your great delight and benefit.

Emmanuel

Faith is courage;

it is creative while despair is always destructive.

David S. Muzzey

Hope springs exulting on triumphant wing.

Robert Burns

Hope is some extraordinary spiritual grace

that God gives us to control our fears,

not to oust them.

Vincent McNabb

Life without faith in something

is too narrow a space to live.

George Lancaster Spalding

We should not let our fears hold us back

from pursuing our hopes.

John F. Kennedy

Hope never abandons you,

you abandon it.

George Weinberg

Tell you the truth,

if you have faith as small as a mustard seed,

you can say to this mountain,

"Move from here to there", and it will move.

Nothing will be impossible to you.

Matthew 17:20

Some see a hopeless end,

while others see an endless hope.

Anonymous

I have found that if you love life,

life will love you back.

Arthur Rubinstein

Seek out that particular mental attribute

which makes you feel most deeply and vitally alive,

along with which comes the inner voice which says,

'This is the real me',

and when you have found that attitude,

follow it.

William James

Hope is the poor man's bread.

Gary Herbert

There is no hope unmingled with fear,

and no fear unmingled with hope.

Baruch Spinoza

Some people are always grumbling

because roses have thorns;

I am thankful

that thorns have roses.

Alphonse Karr

Hopes are but the dreams of those that wake.

Mathew Prior

HAPPINESS

Living a Joyous and Fulfilling Life

You're alive! Be happy! You get to breathe the air, be with friends and family, and enjoy all the glorious wonders of this world. Surviving death can bring you new life; make it a happy one.

Being happy doesn't mean everything is perfect.

It means you have decided

to look beyond the imperfections.

Anonymous

In order to have great happiness

you have to have great pain and unhappiness –

otherwise how would you know when you're happy?

Leslie Caron

Happiness resides not in possessions and not in gold;

the feeling of happiness dwells in the soul.

Democritus

There is no value in life except

what you choose to place upon it

and no happiness in any place except

what you bring to it yourself.

Henry David Thoreau

A cloudy day is no match for a sunny disposition.

William Arthur Ward

Plenty of people miss their share of happiness,

not because they never found it,

but because they didn't stop to enjoy it.

William Feather

Often people attempt to live their lives backwards;

they try to have more things, or more money,

in order to do more of what they want,

so they will be happier.

The way it actually works is the reverse.

You must first be who you really are,

then do what you need to do,

in order to have what you want.

Margaret Young

We tend to forget that happiness doesn't come

as a result of getting something we don't have,

but rather of recognizing and appreciating

what we do have.

Frederick Keonig

Pleasure is spread through the earth.

In stray gifts to be claimed by whoever shall find.

William Wordsworth

Happiness is in the heart,

not in the circumstances.

Anonymous

Enjoy the little things,

for one day you may look back

and realize they were the big things.

Robert Brault

People take different roads seeking

fulfillment and happiness.

Just because they're not on your road

doesn't mean they've gotten lost.

H. Jackson Browne

Happiness often sneaks in through a door

you didn't know you left open.

John Barrymore

Man must search for what is right,

and let happiness come on its own.

Johann Pestalozzi

Happiness is when what you think,

what you say, and what you do

are in harmony.

Mahatma Gandhi

When you're really happy,

the birds chirp and the sun shines

even on cold dark winter nights –

and flowers will bloom on a barren land.

Grey Livingston

Three grand essentials to happiness in this life are

something to do,

something to love,

and something to hope for.

Joseph Addison

One filled with joy

preaches without preaching.

Mother Teresa

Most folks are about as happy

as they make up their minds to be.

Abraham Lincoln

Even if happiness forgets you a little bit,

never completely forget about it.

Jacques Prévert

The happiness of life is made up of minute fractions –

the little soon-forgotten charities of a kiss,

a smile, a kind look, a heartfelt compliment

in the disguise of a playful raillery,

and the countless other infinitesimals

of pleasurable thought and genial feeling.

Samuel Taylor Coleridge

Man is fond of counting his troubles,

but he does not count his joys.

If he counted them up as he ought to,

he would see that every lot

has enough happiness provided for it.

Fyodor Dostoevsky

Happiness is a direction, not a place.

Sydney J. Harris

A truly happy person is one

who can enjoy the scenery while on a detour.

Anonymous

Happiness is not a matter of intensity

but of balance, order, rhythm and harmony.

Thomas Merton

No man is happy

who does not think himself so.

Publilius Syrus

Joy is not in things;

it is in us.

Richard Wagner

Happiness is not a matter of events,

it depends upon the tides of the mind.

Alice Meynell

Happiness or unhappiness

is often a matter of choice.

Anonymous

It makes no difference where you go,

there you are.

And it makes no difference what you have,

there's always more to want.

Until you are happy with who you are,

you will never be happy because of what you have.

Zig Ziglar

If you want to be happy, be.

Leo Tolstoy

The foolish man seeks happiness in the distance;

the wise grows it under his feet.

James Openheim

On the whole, the happiest people seem to be those

who have no particular cause for being happy

except that they are so.

William R. Inge

One joy scatters a hundred griefs.

Chinese Proverb

The rays of happiness,

like those of light,

are colorless when unbroken.

Henry Wadsworth Longfellow

It takes seventy-two muscles to frown,

but only thirteen to smile.

Anonymous

Hope is itself a species of happiness and, perhaps,

the chief happiness which this world affords.

Samuel Johnson

Cheerfulness is what greases the axles of the world.

Don't go through life creaking.

H.W. Byles

When one door of happiness closes, another opens,

but often we look so long at the closed door

that we do not see the one that has been opened for us.

Helen Keller

Happiness is a function of accepting what is.

Werner Erhard

Happiness depends

more on the inward disposition of mind

than on outward circumstances.

Benjamin Franklin

If you ever find happiness by hunting for it,

you will find it,

as the old woman did her lost spectacles,

safe on her own nose all the time.

Josh Billings

Joy is a flower

that blooms when you do.

Anonymous

Happiness is an attitude.

We either make ourselves miserable, or happy and strong.

The amount of work is the same.

Francesca Reigler

Let us be grateful to people who make us happy,

they are the charming gardeners

who make our souls blossom.

Marcel Proust

To be without some of the things you want

is an indispensable part of happiness.

Bertrand Russell

Happiness cannot be traveled to,

owned, earned, worn or consumed.

Happiness is the spiritual experience

of living every minute

with love, grace and gratitude.

Denis Waitley

The art of living does not consist

in preserving and clinging

to a particular mode of happiness,

but in allowing happiness to change its form

without being disappointed by the change;

happiness, like a child, must be allowed to grow up.

Charles L. Morgan

Happiness is not a state to arrive at,

but a manner of traveling.

Margaret Lee Runbeck

There is only one person

who could ever make you happy,

and that person is you.

David Burns

Happiness makes up in height

for what it lacks in length.

Robert Frost

If you want others to be happy,

practice compassion.

If you want to be happy,

practice compassion.

Dalai Lama

There is only one way to happiness,

and that is to cease worrying about things

which are beyond the power of our will.

Epictetus

There is no cosmetic for beauty like happiness.

Lady Blessington

Happiness is a conscious choice,

not an automatic response.

Mildred Barthel

Happiness is a form of courage.

Holbrook Jackson

Happiness always looks small

while you hold it in your hands, but let it go,

and you learn at once how big and precious it is.

Maxim Gorky

Some pursue happiness,

others create it.

Anonymous

Happiness grows at our own firesides,

and is not to be picked in strangers' gardens.

Douglas Jerrold

Knowledge of what is possible

is the beginning of happiness.

George Santayana

Happiness pulses

with every beat of my heart.

Emily Logan Decens

People don't notice

whether it's winter or summer

when they're happy.

Anton Chekhov

A day without laughter is a day wasted.

Charlie Chaplin

I must accept life unconditionally.

Most people ask for happiness on condition.

Happiness can only be felt

if you don't set any condition.

Margaret Lee Runbeck

HARMONY

Finding Internal Peace and Balance

Each survivor will choose to deal with cancer in his or her our own way. Yet, all desire for that moment during recovery when he or she can let go, move on, and finally feel a sense of relief. Every breast cancer survivor wants to make peace with his or her cancer. The search for this peace is inside of you.

Peace of mind is that mental condition in which

you have accepted the worst.

Lin Yn-tang

When there is harmony between

the mind, heart and resolution

then nothing is impossible.

Rig Veda

For every minute you remain angry,

you give up sixty seconds of peace of mind.

Ralph Waldo Emerson

You'll never find peace of mind

until you listen to your heart.

George Michael

He who lives in harmony with himself

lives in harmony with the universe.

Marcus Aurelius

Every goal, every action, every thought,

every feeling one experiences,

whether it be consciously or unconsciously known,

is an attempt to increase

one's level of peace of mind.

Sidney Madwed

Do not believe in anything simply because

you have heard it.

Do not believe in anything simply because

it is spoken and rumored by many.

Do not believe in anything simply because

it is found written in your religious books.

Do not believe in anything merely

on the authority of your teachers and elders.

Do not believe in traditions because

they have been handed down for many generations.

But after observation and analysis,

when you find that anything agrees with reason

and is conducive to the good and benefit of one and all,

then accept it and live up to it.

Buddha

The privilege of a lifetime

is being who you are.

Joseph Campbell

Holding on to anger is like grasping a hot coal

with the intent of throwing it at someone else;

you are the one getting burned.

Buddha

Spirit is an invisible force made visible in all life.

Maya Angelou

What we achieve inwardly

will change outer reality.

Otto Rank

Part of being a healthy person is being

well integrated and at peace.

Candace Pert

You must enshrine in your hearts the spiritual urge

towards light and love, Wisdom and Bliss.

Sri Sathya Sai Baba

A peace above all earthly dignities,

a still and quiet conscience.

William Shakespeare

Let the tears flow of their own accord:

their flowing is not inconsistent

with inward peace and harmony.

Seneca

Nothing can bring you peace but yourself.

Ralph Waldo Emerson

Do not overrate what you have received,

nor envy others.

He who envies others

does not obtain peace of mind.

Buddha

Until you make peace with who you are,

you'll never be content with what you have.

Doris Mortman

When you've seen beyond yourself,

then you may find,

peace of mind is waiting there.

George Harrison

You have to acquire a personal peace of mind

which comes with understanding.

Sandy Woodward

A smile is the beginning of peace.

Mother Teresa

Always aim at

complete harmony of thought and word and deed.

Always aim at

purifying your thoughts and everything will be well.

Mahatma Gandhi

It isn't until you come to a

spiritual understanding of who you are –

not necessarily a religious feeling,

but deep down, the spirit within –

that you can begin to take control.

Oprah Winfrey

All God wants of man is a peaceful heart.

Meister Eckhart

Every person, all the events of your life,

are there because you have drawn them there.

What you choose to do with them is up to you.

Richard Bach

Peace comes from within.

Do not seek it without.

Buddha

There are many things that are essential

to arriving at true peace of mind,

and one of the most important is faith.

John Wooden

When we are present in each moment,

the past gently rolls up behind us

and the future slowly unravels before us.

Rev Richard Levy

Set peace of mind as your highest goal,

and organize your life around it.

Brian Tracy

Dedicate yourself to the

good you deserve and desire for yourself.

Give yourself peace of mind.

You deserve to be happy.

You deserve delight.

Hannah Arendt

Let loose of what you can't control.

Serenity will be yours.

Anonymous

True peace is found in this moment.

Acceptance is the first step to inner calm.

Anonymous

However, when we shift our awareness

or "frequency" from self-consciousness –

where fear, impossibility or feelings of separation reside –

to cosmic consciousness,

which is in total harmony with the universe

and where none of those feelings exist,

then anything is possible.

Rhonda Byrne

Affirm divine calmness and peace,

and send out only thoughts of love and goodwill

if you want to live in peace and harmony.

Never get angry, for anger poisons your system.

Paramahansa Yogananda

For peace of mind,

resign as general manager of the universe.

Larry Eisenberg

Give up what appears to be doubtful for what is certain.

Truth brings peace of mind, and deception doubt.

Muhammad Ali

Peace of mind happens to a man

only after he has developed deep insight,

only after he starts seeing the things

in the right perspective.

Sam Veda

Inner peace is beyond victory or defeat.

Bhagavad Gita

Without peace of mind,

life is just a shadow of its possibilities.

Jean Borysenko

www.ingramcontent.com/pod-product-compliance
Lightning Source LLC
Chambersburg PA
CBHW030015290326
41934CB00005B/351